# COCONUT TOP TEN

# Coconut Top Ten

*A Fun Guide to Coconut Oil, Coconut
Flour, and Other Coconut Essentials
in Easy-to-Digest Top Ten Lists*

## Morgan H. Bishop

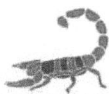

**REDSCORPION**
—PRESS—

# Contents

Introduction   1

1. What Is a Coconut?   5

2. What's Written in the Coconut DNA?   11

3. Ten Shades of Coconuts   15

4. Top Ten Benefits of Coconuts   21

5. Ten Strange Coconut Facts and Uses   31

6. Ten Health and Beauty Uses of Coconut Oil   37

7. Ten Facts About Coconut Water   43

8. Ten Facts About Coconut Sugar   49

9. Ten Coconut Appetizers   53

   Thai Coconut Hummus   53

   Coconut Bites   54

   Coconut Chips   55

   Coconut Energy Bites   56

   Stylish Shrimp Wontons   57

   Crunchy Coconut Apple Bites of Heaven   58

   Nut Bites   58

   Spirulina Coconutty Balls   59

   Coconut Peanut Dip   60

   Quick Deviled Eggs   61

10. Ten Coconut Entrees   63

   Slow-Cooker Coconut Quinoa Curry   63

Chicken Gyro   64

Lentil Coconut Curry   67

Chicken Curry   68

Salmon with Coconut Milk Sauce   70

Creamy Mushroom and Spinach Pasta   71

Beef and Kale Stroganoff   72

Coconut Chicken Fingers   73

Kor-Lae Chicken   74

Chickpea and Spinach Curry   76

11. Ten Coconut Desserts   79

Coconut Dark Chocolate Macaroons   79

Chocolate Coconut Candies   80

Piña Colada Cheesecake   81

Golden Gem Cookies   83

Coconut Triangles   84

Strawberry and Coconut Bars   85

Toasted Coconut Ice Cream   86

Coconut Angel Pie   87

Coconut Hot Chocolate   89

Coconut and Banana Ice Cream   90

12. Ten Coconut Drinks   93

Coconut Beach   93

Cocoa Bliss Smoothie   94

Piña Coladas   94

Coconut Margarita   95

Banana Piña Colada   96

Coconut Rum Slushie   97

Coconut Banana Shake   97

Spicy Coconut Agua Fresca    98

Tropical Water    99

Wild Smoothie    100

Conclusion    103

# Introduction

Are you ready for a coconut adventure? We're going to take you on a journey where you'll discover the amazing world of coconuts. We'll start with the basic facts, and then we'll sail around the world, following the traces written in their genetic code. Along the way, we'll learn why this food has been so highly praised by people all over the world.

In this book you will learn why coconuts are vital for good health and how they can contribute to weight loss. But the benefits don't stop at your waistline. We'll also discuss health benefits such as alleviating acid reflux and increasing levels of potassium and other electrolytes for optimum health.

You will learn about all the forms in which coconuts are found, including water, butter, sugar, vinegar, and oil. All these have their own health benefits and are the reason for the coconut's nickname: "food of the gods."

You will also discover some amazing coconut facts. For example, did you know that coconuts were once used as armor, and that they helped save lives during World War I?

Finally, if you want to make this incredible food part of your diet, we've included a number of delicious recipes that you can easily prepare and enjoy!

## *Why Are Coconuts So Special?*

Coconuts have played a central role in my life from the earliest I can remember. I was weaned on coconut milk . . . which may be why I can now change a flat tire with my bare hands in the rain!

I recall biting into a chocolate-covered macaroon at a champagne and piña colada brunch: I was blown away. Not only does the flavor of coconut drive many people wild (especially when combined with dark rum), but the electrolytes can help vanquish a nasty hangover.

Coconuts are useful beyond their nutritional benefits: my mother would cover her breasts in fresh young coconut shells. As I got older, I realized that she would only wear a brassiere when dignitaries were due to pop in.

I recall the old days of lazing under a regal palm and sipping cool coconut water out of a coconut freshly decapitated by my servant Manny's rusty machete. With coconut water dribbling out of the side of my mouth, I gazed out at the tranquil Caribbean . . .

Coconuts, like the earth, like humans, are at their core, water. But all three are much more than $H_2O$; they all possess as well a divine spirit. I will forever be mesmerized by, and indebted to, the coconut.

# CHAPTER 1
# What Is a Coconut?

The term *coconut* can refer to the entire palm, the fruit, or the seed.

The palm tree's scientific name is *Cocos nucifera*. Together with other palm trees, it belongs to the large Arecaceae family. They are believed to be native to Southeast Asia, where they have been cultivated and used as food for centuries. Coconut palms are generally found in tropical countries, because they require sandy, moist, and well-drained soil. They flourish along the saline-rich coastal regions.

Generally speaking, the coconut palm is a tall tree that can reach a height of more than one hundred feet. Its lifetime can range from seventy-five to a hundred years.[1] Once planted, a coconut tree may need about five years to start producing. One coconut palm may

---

1. "Coconut Palm Trees—Interesting Facts about Them," accessed February 15, 2016, http://www.coconut-info.net/general/coconut_trees.php.

yield from 20 to 150 mature coconuts.[2] The nuts are oval and between five and ten inches wide.

## A Fruit or a Nut?

Is the coconut a fruit or a nut? I was asked the same question when I started wearing smoking jackets crafted from exotic bedsheets . . . but they're just so darn comfortable! This age-old question has been posed about me by both my ex-wives, and once a woman I approached at a bar in Queens said, "So what ah ya? A fruit or a nut?"

There has also been a real debate on the true category of coconuts. Are they a fruit or a nut? Actually, they can be both. Botanically speaking, a coconut is a one-seeded drupe, which belongs to the category of fruits.

A drupe is a fruit which has a hard stony shell that encloses the seed. Drupes include mangos, coffee, dates, olives, almonds, pistachios, cherries, peaches, apricots, nectarines, and plums.[3]

Like all drupes, unhusked coconuts have three

2. "Coconut Palm," accessed February 28, 2016, Encyclopædia Britannica Online, http://www.britannica.com/plant/coconut-palm.

3. "Is Coconut a Fruit or a Nut?" accessed February 17, 2016, http://www.thebestofrawfood.com/is-coconut-a-fruit.html.

layers. The outer layer, the exocarp, is smooth and light green. It turns gray and dry once the nut matures. The middle layer, the mesocarp, is a husk made of tough fibers, and is an inch or two thick. This layer surrounds the woody shell, which is called the endocarp and envelops the edible meat.[4]

Mature coconuts that are recently harvested also contain some amount of sweet liquid in their hollow central cavity. People from non-tropical countries often buy coconuts with the husk removed. The coconut water and the white flesh that we eat is actually the inside of the seed.

A seed is the reproductive part of any flowering plant. Basically, a seed contains two parts: the embryo root and embryo leaves. Now, when you look at a coconut, you will see three pores that are sometimes called eyes. When the coconut seed germinates, a shoot will emerge from one of these pores. Besides this, the seed also contains the food, which will provide the necessary nutrients to support the new life. This food is botanically called the endosperm, and it makes up most of the seed. In the case of coconuts, this is the white stuff that we eat.

Another reason why coconuts can cause confusion (aside from when they are mixed with rum) is because they contain the word *nut* in their name. If we don't rely so much on botanical facts, someone may say that coconuts can be nuts because nuts are defined as a one-seeded fruit. However, coconuts lack other characteristics of nuts. Moreover, coconuts cannot be classified as nuts because they are formed in a different way.

When a coconut is not harvested but is left on the palm, its green outer husk turns brown over time. Then the coconut falls from the tree. If the coconut is left to mature, a green shoot will appear through the husk and shell. The new plant uses the water and white flesh as its food. Eventually, roots will find their way to the soil, where they will gather all the nutrients they need to grow into a tree.

A medium-size coconut has about 400 grams of edible meat and about 30 to 150 milliliters of water.[5] It is also rich in saturated fats, the most important of which is lauric acid.

5. "Coconuts and Its Secrets—Part I," accessed February 18, 2016, http://www.ecellulitis.com/skin-health/coconuts-and-its-secrets-part-i/.

## Two Coconut Types

There are two types of coconuts, known as *Niu kafa* and *Niu vai*. They differ in shape and color. *Niu kafa*s are triangular, and their husks are large and fibrous. *Niu vai*s are rounder in shape and their color is yellow or bright green. When they are not ripe, they contain sweet coconut water.[6]

When I'm too ripe, I've noticed that people do not like to stand in my vicinity. Perhaps they would come closer if I smelled more like a coconut.

---

6. "Deep History of Coconuts Decoded," Diana Lutz, Washington University in Saint Louis, last modified June 24, 2011, accessed February 20, 2016, https://source.wustl.edu/2011/06/deep-history-of-coconuts-decoded/.

# CHAPTER 2
# What's Written in the Coconut DNA?

The term *coconut* can be traced back to the sixteenth century and the Spanish word *coco*, which means "a monkey face" or "a grin." This probably comes from the fact that a husked coconut slightly resembles a monkey head or even a human face because of the three indentations called eyes and the hairy shell.

However, the origin of the coconut plant is vague. This truly remarkable food, which is today grown in more than seventy countries around the world, has caused a lot of trouble for those interested in its origin. Scientists have relied on botany, etymology, art, fossils, folklore, and genetics in an attempt to figure out where coconuts appeared for the first time.

There has been a lengthy debate on whether coconuts came from the Old World or the New World. (One thing for sure: when mixed with a cacophony of booze, as in a coco-loco, they are *out* of this world!) At the beginning of the twentieth century, a palm specialist, Odoardo Beccari (not to be confused with Ron Bacardi), claimed that the coconut came from the Old World, more precisely from Polynesia or the Indian Archipelago. He supported his claim by pointing out that the Eastern Hemisphere has more varieties of coconut palm than North and South America. (Not to mention more varieties of Chinese food and massage parlors.)

Another group of scientists, including K. F. P. von Martius, H. B. Guppy, and O. F. Cook, believed that coconuts were from the New World and then found their way west across the Pacific Ocean.[7]

There has been one major study led by a group of researchers and evolutionary botanists determined to break the coconut DNA code. The research, which included more than 1,300 coconuts from all over the world, was conducted at Washington University.[8]

---

7. "Is a Coconut a Fruit, Nut or Seed?" accessed February 19, 2016, The Library of Congress, http://www.loc.gov/rr/scitech/mysteries/coconut.html.

8. Gunn, B. F. et al. "Independent Origins of Cultivated Coconut (Cocos nucifera L.) in the Tropics," PLoS ONE 6 no. 3 (2011): e21143 DOI:10.1371/journal.pone.0021143.

The findings indicated that the coconut had two places of origin: the Indian Ocean basin and the Pacific basin. However, what is written in the coconut DNA is not only its origin, but also the records of exploration and colonization. It's really amazing how the history of people is interwoven with the history of coconuts.

This group of scientists, led by Kenneth Olsen, analyzed the DNA of both Pacific and Indian Ocean coconuts, and discovered that these two types are genetically different. This was an amazing discovery because, after all, these two types of coconuts belong to the same species. This served as evidence that the coconut had two origins of cultivation.

Another remarkable discovery concerns the coconuts from the Comoros Islands and Madagascar. They form an exception to this split between the two types of coconuts and represent a genetic mixture of the two types.

But how did the coconut migrate?

The team of researchers believes that ancient Austronesians introduced Pacific coconuts to the Indian Ocean region several thousand years ago. These people had established trade routes that allowed both them and coconuts to travel.

Later, the coconut found its way to Europeans, who brought it to the New World. That's why a majority of coconuts found in Florida today are of the Indian Ocean type. The reason for the number of bored retirees in the Sunshine State is still a mystery. But I wish they would leave me alone!

The coconut has a special place in Indian mythology and rituals, indicating its importance for the region. There's a reason it's called the fruit of the gods. Even today, coconuts remain a revered part of Indian culture and are known as one of the essential resources, not only for food but also for fuel, shelter, and tools. (And, thank God, for bras.)

Nowadays, the coconut is found in dishes and cocktails all over the world, not only because of its delectable flavor and aroma but also because of its health benefits. Its health-promoting properties have also been recognized by the cosmetics industry, and coconut can be found in scrubs, creams, lotions, and a variety of other products.

# CHAPTER 3
# Ten Shades of Coconuts

## 1. Coconut Water

Coconut water is the liquid that is found inside young coconuts. It contains electrolytes and potassium, and is revered by athletes because of its hydrating properties. For those who prefer to drink alcohol athletically, there's good news: it's also great for hangovers!

Coconut water is cool and crisp. It consists of electrolytes, simple sugars, minerals, bioactive compounds such as cytokine, and enzymes such as catalase, phosphatase, polymerases, and dehydrogenase peroxidase. It is a good source of minerals and vitamins, and has found its place in many healthy diets.

## 2. Coconut Milk

To make coconut milk, coconut meat is blended with water and then strained. The quality and fat content varies by brand, but you can always make your own coconut milk at home. It will take you just a few minutes. Blend the water and meat on high in your blender, and then strain the milk. More notes on turning this stuff into piña coladas later.

### 3. Coconut Cream

Coconut cream is what separates from canned coconut milk once it is left in the fridge for a while. You will notice that the cream floats to the top. You can use it instead of whipped cream. Though it may seem like exactly the same thing as coconut butter, it is not. Unlike coconut butter, it does not contain fiber and is strained.

### 4. Coconut Flakes

These are basically small morsels of dried coconut meat. You can toast them and use them as a snack or make some DIY coconut butter or milk.

### 5. Coconut Flour

Coconut flour is also dried coconut, but it is ground so that it contains the whole fiber content. Those on a gluten-free diet use this flour as a substitute for wheat or other flours. However, due to its fiber content, it acts as a powerful absorbent, soaking up the moisture from cakes and batters. When adapting recipes for coconut flour, the rule of thumb is to use a quarter cup of coconut flour for one cup of white flour.

## 6. Coconut Oil

Coconut oil is actually the pure fat that comes from the coconut meat. There are a few varieties of coconut oil, which are distinguished by the processing method.[9]

- Virgin—raw coconut meat is used, and it is not heated. It tends to taste quite innocent.
- Refined—this coconut oil is during the processing method treated with bleaches, deodorizers, and other chemicals. It doesn't have the coconut taste and smell that virgin coconut oil has. Prefers bold red wine and Daniel Day-Lewis movies.
- Unrefined—has a strong coconut flavor as it is

---

9. "Raw, Virgin, Unrefined, Organic, Expeller-Pressed Coconut Oil—Which Is Best?" last modified February 25, 2009, http://kellythekitchenkop.com/raw-virgin-unrefined-organic-expeller-pressed-coconut-oil-which-is-best/.

not treated with chemicals. Virgin coconut oil falls into this category. Tends to enjoy wine coolers and anything with Tom Green.

- Expeller-pressed—coconut oil obtained from the manual pressing of the coconut meat, not by using chemicals. Expeller-pressed oil is generally humorless.

## 7. Coconut Sugar

Coconut sugar is also known as coconut crystals or coconut nectar. Although there are many who think of coconut sugar as a superfood, it is rich in calories and cannot do wonders as many may expect. It is true that it is somewhat healthier than cane sugar, but you should limit your intake. Unfortunately, the same rules apply to coconut rum.

## 8. Coconut Butter

You can find coconut butter under the name coconut cream concentrate. Coconut butter is made by grinding the meat into a pulp. The result is a substance much finer than coconut flour. It can be used like any other nut butter. When you buy a jar of coconut butter, you'll notice that it is separated into two layers—the oil and meat. You just need to melt it and combine them. Coconut peanut butter (which is peanut butter made with coconut oil) is also delicious, and much more nutritious than name-brand peanut butter.

## 9. Coconut Aminos

Coconut aminos is made from the coconut sap, which is then combined with salt. This product is mostly used in the paleo diet as a substitute for soy sauce.

## 10. Coconut Vinegar

Coconut vinegar is made from fermenting coconut sap. It is white and cloudy, and has an acidic flavor resembling that of balsamic or apple-cider vinegar. It can be substituted for other vinegars in many recipes, with tasty results.

# CHAPTER 4
# Top Ten Benefits of Coconuts

For many years, coconuts have been wrongly accused of being a food to avoid if you want to stay healthy. This is one of the major ways that I empathize with coconuts. I too have been wrongly accused of many things, and some people have stopped hanging out with me as a result. In the case of coconuts, the crime was primarily their high saturated-fat content. However, recent studies have proven that the fat content actually comes from medium-chain triglycerides. These elements go to the liver, which means that there are very few MCTs left to deposit in fat tissues. So, instead of piling on, they are burned off as energy.[10]

The risk of stroke and other heart diseases among the Tokelaus of New Zealand and Kitavans of Papua New Guinea is much lower than in Western coun-

10 "Beneficial Effects on Energy, Atherosclerosis and Aging," Ward Dean and Jim English, Nutritionre, last modified April 22, 2013, accessed February 23, 2016, http://nutritionreview.org/2013/04/medium-chain-triglycerides

tries.[11] The key to the health of these people may lie in the fact that coconuts are their staple food. Coconuts are nowadays widely available, so that all can enjoy their benefits. The benefits mentioned and discussed here have all been scientifically confirmed, so know that you are in good hands.

## 1. Helps You Stay Young

Many people who wish to stay young eat coconuts because of their antioxidant content. This is why my conditional driver's license says I am in my sixties but I don't look a day over forty-two (okay, fifty-two). Antioxidants have proven to be successful in protecting the body and cells from the damaging effects of free radicals that our bodies produce. The damage these free radicals cause can have numerous negative consequences, including the increased risk of developing cancer.

## 2. Helps You Regenerate After a Workout

Coconut water has become popular as a natural hydrator, as it contains electrolytes, which are important for

11. "The Kitavan Diet: Tubers, Fresh Fruit, Coconut and Fish," accessed February 19, 2016, http://www.healwithfood.org/diet/kitavan-diet-foods.php#ixzz41TyA18hu.

the function of our muscles and nerves. Coconut water also appears to be great for light workouts, because your body loses potassium through sweat. A cup of coconut water contains more than 10 percent of the daily recommended dose of this mineral. Though I understand that this "working out" thing is beneficial, I have not yet tried it. I get my exercise the old-fashioned way: I earn it.

Another great thing that makes coconut water a good option after a workout is that it is fat free and contains low amounts of carbs, calories, and sugars. Moreover, it has high amounts of B vitamins, ascorbic acid, and proteins.[12]

## 3. Reduces Symptoms of Alzheimer's Disease

The fats coconut oil contains are almost 90 percent fatty acids that are saturated. New data indicate that saturated fats have nothing to do with clogging arteries and being harmful to human health. Coconut oil is rich in medium-chain triglycerides (MCTs). These fatty acids are metabolized differently from long-chain fatty acids. When these fatty acids enter the digestive system, they immediately go to the liver. Here, they

---

12. "The Truth about Coconut Water," Kathleen M. Zelman, accessed February 28, 2016, http://www.webmd.com/food-recipes/truth-about-coconut-water.

are turned into the so-called ketone bodies or are used as a quick source of energy. This, in turn, has beneficial effects on some brain disorders such as Alzheimer's and epilepsy.[13]

An increased risk of Alzheimer's disease has been observed in elderly individuals. It has been found out that those suffering from this disease can't use glucose for energy in certain parts of the brain. Ketone bodies are also known to supply the brain with energy. These ketones are possibly an alternative source of energy for the malfunctioning cells that cause Alzheimer's.

A study of patients whose Alzheimer's symptoms were not severe indicated that consumption of MCTs can improve the brain function.[14] This study motivated other researchers to intensively study these potential therapeutic effects of coconut oil on reducing the symptoms of Alzheimer's disease.

The ketogenic diet, based on very low carb and high fat intake, can treat various health disorders. This diet is praised for reducing epilepsy seizures in children, particularly those cases in which epilepsy is drug resistant. Since the MCTs found in coconut oil go

13. Phan, N. "Ketogenic Diet as a Treatment for Refractory Epilepsy," *Journal on Developmental Disabilities* 13 no. 3 (2007): 187–204.

14. Costantini, L. et al. "Hypometabolism as a Therapeutic Target in Alzheimer's Disease," *BMC Neuroscience* 9 no. 2 (2008): S16.

straight to the liver, where they are turned into ketone bodies, there is potential to use them in epileptic patients to induce ketosis.

## 4. Fights Candida

The acids in coconut oil can help eliminate the bacteria that cause candida.[15]

## 5. Helps You Lose Weight

Obesity is one of the most common underlying causes of health problems. Most people think that simply taking in lots of calories leads to gaining weight. However, the source of these calories is important as well. The reason is obvious: various foods affect our bodies differently. Not every calorie you take in behaves the same way; it may not even be counted as a calorie. For instance, medium-chain triglycerides have been shown to increase energy expenditure when compared to the same amount of calories that come from longer-chain fats.

Coconut oil is particularly beneficial for reducing abdominal fat, which lodges around organs in the

---

15. "Health Benefits of Coconut Oil," accessed February 27, 2016, https://www.organicfacts.net/health-benefits/oils/health-benefits-of-coconut-oil.html.

abdominal cavity. This kind of fat is very dangerous because it is associated with many modern diseases. Your waistline is a clear indicator of the amount of abdominal fat.

A study of forty women with abdominal obesity who were instructed to take in one ounce of coconut oil per day showed that this caused a significant drop in both waist circumference and body mass over the period of a year.[16] Exercise was not included in this study, and the intake of calories was not restricted, so the results were impressive.

Another way in which coconut oil can help you reduce weight is by reducing your hunger. This is actually related to the fact that these fatty acids are metabolized differently and are turned into ketone bodies, which can reduce appetite.[17]

The results of several studies show that a short-term influence of coconut oil on losing weight is significant, and in the long run it can lead to a balanced weight loss.

16. Assunção, M. L. et al. "Effects of Dietary Coconut Oil on the Biochemical and Anthropometric Profiles of Women Presenting Abdominal Obesity," Lipids 44 no. 7 (2009): 593–601.

17. McClernon, F. J. et al. "The Effects of a Low-Carbohydrate Ketogenic Diet and a Low-Fat Diet on Mood, Hunger, and Other Self-Reported Symptoms," Obesity (Silver Spring) 15 no. 1 (2007): 182–187.

## 6. Improves Digestion

Coconuts, and particularly coconut oil, aid in digestion because they help the body absorb amino acids, minerals, and vitamins. The saturated fats give coconut oil its antimicrobial properties. It can also soothe some of the burning caused by acid reflux.[18]

## 7. Lowers Risk of Heart Disease

Coconut oil is rich in saturated fats, which are not as harmful as was once thought. These fats have been shown to raise HDL, known as the good cholesterol, but they also turn the LDL cholesterol into its benign subtype.

Studies have proven that coconut oil can reduce total and LDL cholesterol, while at the same time increasing HDL cholesterol.[19, 20] In the long run, these benefits can lead to a reduced risk of heart disease. However, some scientists suggest that coconut oil

18. Shilhavy, Brian and Marianita. "Coconut Oil Benefits for Digestive Health," accessed February 29, 2016, http://healthimpactnews.com/20012/coconut-oil-benefits-for-digestive-health/.

19. Dreaon, D. M. et al. "Change in Dietary Saturated Fat Intake is Correlated with Change in Mas of Large *Low-Density-Lipoprotein Particles in Men,*" American Journal of Clinical Nutrition 67 no. 5 (1998): 828–836.

20. Nevin, K. G., and Rajamohan, T. "Influence of Virgin Coconut Oil on Blood Coagulation Factors, Lipid Levels and LDL Oxidation in Cholesterol Fed Sprague-Dawley Rats," European *e-Journal of Clinical Nutrition and Metabolistm* 3 no. 1 (2008): e1–e8.

should be used in moderation.

Coconut milk can also be beneficial for heart health. It is a good source of vitamins E and A, as well as phytosterols and polyphenols. All these elements work together to decrease LDL cholesterol. This cholesterol actually refers to the fats that stay in the blood and skin tissues. These have been recognized as one of the leading causes of cardiovascular diseases.

## 8. Adds Fiber to Your Diet and Is Diabetes-Safe

Coconut flour can add that recognizable coconutty flavor to your meals. It is also great for adding fiber. Two tablespoons of coconut flour deliver five grams of fiber and only two grams of fat.

People suffering from diabetes can also benefit from coconut flour, because it reduces the glycemic index.

## 9. Boosts Your Metabolism

Coconuts have antibacterial, antifungal, and antiviral properties. It is no wonder that they can strengthen our immune system. All these properties come from lauric acid, antimicrobial lipids, caprylic acid, and capric acid. When lauric acid enters the body, it gets converted into monolaurin, which studies indicate helps to protect the body from bacteria and viruses.

## 10. Beauty Benefits

If coconuts were not so beneficial for our health and beauty, there wouldn't be so many cosmetic products that include coconuts. Coconuts have proven particularly efficacious in making hair shiny and lustrous. Furthermore, it has been observed that coconut water reduced excessive skin oil and can alleviate acne and other skin blemishes. I have also been experimenting with coconut beard oil, essentially rubbing liquid coconut oil into my beard, with some glistening results.

# CHAPTER 5
# Ten Strange Coconut Facts and Uses

Yes, it is a delicious food, and great for cocktails and beards, but the coconut has other uses, some of which will surely surprise you. Here are a few little-known facts from the vaults.

## 1. Coconut Gas Masks

During World War I, when the concept of gas warfare was developed, gas masks became necessary. Basically, to scrub the air clean, gas masks make use of carbon. However, there are different types of carbon. Gas mask manufacturers in the United States discovered that gas masks using coconut-fiber carbon were more efficacious than gas masks that used other filtering substances. This carbon, which is obtained by burning coconut husks, is still considered an important element in cleaning up radiation. It was even used during the cleanup at the Fukushima nuclear plant.[21]

## 2. Coconut Crafts

Artists all over the world find creative ways to show off their talents. Coconut makes a good material for sculptures, and it can also serve as a canvas for gifted artists. I like to make bizarre faces on my discarded coconuts, creating tropical jack o' lanterns.

## 3. Drums for Folk Dances

The maglalatik is a dance indigenous to the Philippines in which men attach coconut halves to their bodies. As they dance, the coconut halves clap and produce a drum-like sound.

## 4. Coconut Fuel

Peanut oil was used to run early combustion-engine machines, and coconut oil can be used as fuel as well.[22]

21. "10 Awesome Facts About Coconuts," Patrick Icasas, last modified August 28, 2013, accessed February 18, 2016, http://listverse.com/2013/08.28/ 10-awesome-facts-about-coconuts/.

22. "Biofuel," accessed February 20, 2016, http://www.kokonutpacific.com.au/CoconutBiofuelKP.php#continued.

It is a planet-friendly alternative to fossil fuels because coconut trees are able to produce oil in workable quantities. It can be used as a substitute for petroleum diesel and can also serve as an additive or base substance.

## 5. Coconut Armor

No, this is not a hollowed-out coconut husk that you use as a helmet. Coconut armor is much more than that. Get ready for this. In the small Micronesian archipelago of Kiribati, skilled craftsmen used to make a true coconut armor, consisting of body armor, cap, jerkin, leggings, and back plate.[23] They used coconut fiber, which was woven so densely that the armor resembled a kind of thick carpet. To this day, I wear coconut armor into battle.

## 6. Coconut Plasma

Coconut water can be used as a substitute for human blood plasma.[24]

23. "10 Awesome Facts About Coconuts," Patrick Icasas, last modified August 28, 2013, accessed February 18, 2016, http://listverse.com/2013/08.28/ 10-awesome-facts-about-coconuts/.

24. Campbell-Falck, D. et al. (2000). "The Intravenous Use of Coconut Water. *American Journal of Emergency Medicine* 18, no. 1: 108–11.

Of course, this is just a short-term solution . . . but so is the U.S. social security system. The plasma was tested back in the 1950s, when it was used to treat a severely dehydrated patient from the Solomon Islands. As a side note, rum doesn't work.

## 7. Building Materials

Thanks to their lignin content, which acts as a natural adhesive, coconut husks can be used for producing high-quality board materials. The production does not involve the addition of chemical binders or glues.

In this process, the coconut flesh and fibers are separated, and after being processed into small pieces, the husk undergoes intense heated pressure and is formed into boards called ecoco boards. Thus, something that would otherwise be dumped is used for producing useful materials.

## 8. Coconet

Coconut husks find a large array of uses because they are resistant to salt water and don't break down easily. An inventor from the Philippines found an interesting way to use coconut-husk fibers. He created nets that are biodegradable and are used on riverbanks and sloping land, thus increasing plant growth and protecting against erosion.[25]

## 9. Substitute for Synthetic Fibers

Researchers from Baylor University found a way to use coconut fibers instead of synthetic fibers in the production of some car parts.[26] These fibers are mostly used for floorboards, bed liners, inside door covers, and in sun visors.

## 10. Fertilizer

Coconut husks can be used as a fertilizer to grow mushrooms and orchids. Coconut-husk ash is used because it is rich in potassium. In a recent study, mature coconut palms that were fertilized with coconut-husk ash showed greater yield than palms from the control group.[27]

25. "Coconets," last modified April 27, 2012, accessed February 2, 2016, http://www.aljazeera.com/programmes/earthrise/2012/04.201242715330787850.html

26. "Company Converts Coconut Husk Fibers into Materials for Cars and Homes," Marlene Cimons, last modified July 23, 2014, accessed February 21, 2016, http://phys.org/news/2014-07-company-coconut-husk-fibers-materials.html.

27. Bonneau, X. et al. "Coconut Husk Ash as a Fertilizer for Coconut Palms on Peat," *Experimental Agriculture* 46 no. 3 (2010): 401-414.

# CHAPTER 6
# Ten Health and Beauty Uses of Coconut Oil

As we have already seen, coconuts are highly versatile. Maybe you already use coconut oil in your kitchen, but did you know that coconuts can be used for the purposes of health and beauty as well? Here, you'll find ways to include coconuts in your beauty routine.

## 1. Hair Mask

Coconut oil is a creamy substance that turns into liquid when heated to 76 degrees Fahrenheit. It is great for giving your hair (or beard) a shine, as well as moisturizing and repairing it. To make a hair mask, just hold the jar containing coconut oil under warm water. When the oil melts, generously apply the oil to wet strands of hair. If your hair is long enough, twist it into a bun. Leave it in for at least five minutes and then rinse.

You can even make a shampoo. It is chemical-free and is made of just two ingredients—coconut oil and apple-cider vinegar. This shampoo makes your hair shiny and soft and prevents yellow and orange discoloration.

## 2. Body Oil

Coconut oil contains antioxidants and vitamins that keep the skin healthy and moisturized. Apply it to your skin after a shower while your skin is still warm. This will melt the oil so that it will sink into your skin. Coconut oil is not greasy, and the skin absorbs it quickly. Plus, it will give your skin that alluring tropical scent.

## 3. Under-Eye Cream

Coconut oil is also beneficial for keeping the delicate skin area under your eyes silky and young-looking. Since the skin under your eyes is very thin, chances are that dark circles and fine lines will appear here more often. To treat this area with coconut oil, just apply a pinch of it, but first rub it between your fingers to warm it up. There's no need to spend a fortune on expensive creams and lotions when you can use coconut oil.

## 4. Makeup Remover

It may sound surprising, but coconut oil can help you remove your makeup easily. Just apply warmed coconut oil to your skin and massage it in nicely, and you'll see how it all melts away. Then simply rinse your skin with warm water.

You can even create makeup-remover wipes. For this, you will need a teaspoon of melted coconut for each cotton pad. Add the cotton pads to the liquefied coconut oil and leave them to soak overnight. You can store these in a plastic baggie. They are great for removing makeup from your eyes because coconut oil will not irritate your eyes or sting them.

Although I don't wear as much makeup as I once did, coconut oil gives me the confidence that I can get it off in a hurry if I need to.

## 5. Body Scrub

To prepare a scrub that moisturizes your skin and makes it smooth by removing dead skin cells, you will need only two basic ingredients: a cup of melted coconut oil and a cup of sugar or sea salt. If your skin, elbows, or feet are tough, just add more sugar or salt and buff away.

## 6. Teeth Health

To whiten your teeth, freshen your breath, and improve gum health, make a mixture of equal parts baking soda and coconut oil. Add a few drops of peppermint essential oil. Research conducted at the Athlone Institute of technology indicated that, thanks to its antibiotic properties, coconut oil can destroy bacteria in the mouth that cause tooth decay.[28]

Another way to use coconut oil for keeping your teeth healthy is to do coconut oil pulling. After you get up in the morning, swish a tablespoon of coconut oil in your mouth for ten to twenty minutes. Make sure you don't swallow the oil. Spit the oil into your trashcan and rinse your mouth with sea-salt water. This will protect your teeth from decay, kill bad breath, and detoxify your mouth. This method of keeping your mouth and teeth healthy is culled from Ayurvedic medicine.

---

28 "Coconut Oil Could Combat Tooth Decay," last modified September 3, 2012, accessed February 21, 2016, BBC, http://www.bbc.com/news/health-19435442.

## 7. Wound Salve

Because of its antifungal and antibacterial properties, coconut oil can be used as first aid in treating burns, rashes, and open wounds. A mixture of coconut oil, lavender, frankincense, and melaleuca oil can be used to speed healing of skin after infections. It is also recognized as one of the best natural sunburn remedies.

## 8. Cellulite and Stretch-Mark Reducer

Stretch marks have plagued me for years. But I am proud to say that I remain cellulite free. For those dealing with these unsightly issues, coconut is a magic elixir. With coconut oil, you can finally see results in getting rid of that stubborn cellulite. Prepare a mixture of ten drops of grapefruit essential oil and a tablespoon of coconut oil. Use this mixture to massage the affected areas, using firm circular motions. To encourage cellular detox after a massage, you can finish with dry brushing, which will stimulate circulation.

Rub coconut oil over your stomach both during and after pregnancy. This will reduce stretch marks. Your skin will be hydrated and will heal quickly. Also, the coconut oil will reduce the redness, discoloration, and dark marks that occur when the elasticity of the skin is compromised.

## 9. Acne Fighter

Both teenagers and adults can be plagued with acne. The two most common causes of this skin issue are an imbalance in oil on the skin and bacteria overgrowth. But pimples beware! Coconut oil is helpful for treating acne because of its antibiotic properties, which kill the harmful bacteria that lead to this overgrowth. It is particularly beneficial when combined with raw honey and tea tree oil.

## 10. Eczema and Psoriasis Treatment

It is now established that coconut oil does wonders for skin. It is particularly beneficial for dry and flaking skin, and those suffering from psoriasis and eczema find it soothing.[29] For treating these skin problems, coconut oil is most beneficial when combined with geranium oil and shea butter.

29. "Treating Eczema and Psoriasis with Coconut and Other Natural Oils," last modified October 3, 2015, accessed February 22, 2016, http://homeremediesforlife.com/coconut-oil-for-eczema/.

# CHAPTER 7
# Ten Facts About Coconut Water

## 1. Coconut Water Is Super Water

Even though doctors are always haranguing me, I almost never drink water straight. But I make an exception for coconut water. Coconut water is about 95 percent water, which makes it a great hydration drink. During workouts or extended periods of physical activity, the body loses fluids rich in essential minerals. Coconut water is an amazing source of potassium and electrolytes, so it helps you keep your body hydrated. Unlike many other hydrating drinks, it is very low in sugar and doesn't contain nasty preservatives and chemicals.

Coconut water is an amazing source of five electrolytes that are found in the body: magnesium, calcium, potassium, phosphorus, and sodium.[30] Potassium is essential for the nervous system and brain to function properly. And if you feel that your energy level is low, that may be an indication that your body is running low on magnesium. Coconut water has all the rejuvenation powers you need.

## 2. Hangover Remedy

I have extensive experience with hangovers and have tried numerous ways to get rid of them. I can say with confidence that coconut water is one of the best remedies. If you have drunk more than you should have, you should consume coconut water to help you out. Hangovers are often accompanied by vomiting or frequent urination, and this is where coconut water is particularly helpful, because it replaces all those electrolytes that have left your body.

## 3. It's Low in Calories

Coconut water can be an ally in your efforts to lose weight. Since coconut water is low in fat, it can be consumed in large quantities without any fear that you will gain weight, which is not the case with all

30. "Coconut Water Nutrition Facts," accessed February 28, 2016, http://www.nutrition-and-you.com/coconut-water.html.

those sugary drinks. Also, coconut water has been shown to suppress the appetite, which means that it can help in weight-loss efforts.

## 4. Used Instead of Human Plasma

Amazingly, coconut water can be used in emergencies to save people's lives in cases of severe dehydration. It works in place of human plasma if administered intravenously.

## 5. Skin Care

Coconut water is not only super hydrating; it's antibacterial as well. It can alleviate skin blemishes and acne, as it has been shown to moisturize the skin and eliminate excess oil. The cosmetics industry has recognized this property of coconut water, and it can be found in a number of creams and lotions.

## 6. Cooking

Coconut oil may be all the rage when it comes to cooking, but don't overlook coconut water. Since it is a good source of fiber, it goes really well in smoothies. Basically, it can be used in any dish where plain water is used, including doughs, oatmeal, soups, and steamed vegetables.

## 7. Choosing the Right Coconut

The amount of coconut water in coconuts may vary from 200 to 1,000 milliliters. Young coconuts are the best, because they contain a large amount of water. They are ideally used when they are five months old. Younger coconuts may not only be bitter in taste, but also devoid of nutrients. Although mature coconuts contain less water, they are much more sophisticated and responsible.

Choose coconuts that are young and green. Shake the coconut to test how much liquid it contains. (This is a fine art that is coveted in the islands.)

## 8. Aids in Digestion

Since coconut water is a good source of fiber, it can aid in digestion and prevent acid reflux.

## 9. It Contains Cytokinins

Cytokinins are plant growth substances that are plentiful in coconut water. According to recent research, cytokinins can slow the aging process and delay the development of cancerous cells.[31]

## 10. It's Rich in Antioxidants

Coconut water contains plenty of antioxidants, which are known for protecting our bodies from free radicals. Free radicals are the products of our own bodies, which means that there is no other way to fight them unless we consume food rich in antioxidants.

31. "7 More Reasons to Drink Coconut Water," David Brown, last modified April 4, 2015, accessed February 18, 2016, http://mindbodygreen.com/0-18146/7-more-reasons-to-drink-coconut-water.html.

# CHAPTER 8
# Ten Facts About Coconut Sugar

## 1. The Production Process

Coconut sugar is made from coconut flower buds. The fresh sap that oozes out of the flowers when they are cut is collected and then heated until most of the liquid has evaporated. The final stage is drying this mixture in order to remove any residual moisture.

## 2. Taste

Coconut sugar has a pretty brown color, but it doesn't have that distinct coconut flavor. Although its taste is similar to that of brown sugar, it has a more pronounced caramel flavor.

## 3. Variety

Coconut sugar is sold in a variety of forms, such as a soft paste, a syrup, crystals similar to cane sugar, or hard blocks. Coconut sugar is very sticky and dense, even when it is softened.

## 4. Regular Sugar versus Coconut Sugar

Unlike regular sugar, coconut sugar retains most of the nutrients that are found in the coconut palm. According to the Philippine Department of Agriculture, coconut sugar has zinc, iron, potassium, and calcium, as well as amino acids and polyphenols.

## 5. Lowers GI

Coconut sugar contains the fiber called inulin. There are indications that inulin may slow glucose absorption and consequently lower the glycemic index.[32] Foods that have a low glycemic index are beneficial because, after their consumption, there are no spikes in blood-sugar levels.

## 6. Calories and Carbs

Although it is a healthier alternative to regular cane sugar, coconut sugar contains almost the same amount of calories and carbohydrates. The American Diabetes

32. "Coconut Sugar—Healthy Sugar Alternative or a Big, Fat Lie?" Kris Gunnars, last modified November, 2015, accessed February 20, 2016, http// authoritynutrition.com/coconut-sugar/.

Association suggests that people with diabetes should use coconut sugar as a sweetener, but should not think of it as a superfood that is very different from regular sugar.

## 7. Variations in Quality

The quality of coconut sugar varies greatly depending on the age of the tree it is collected from, the type of the tree, and the time of year. Try several varieties to ensure you're getting the finest quality coconut sugar.

## 8. Coconut Sugar Means No Coconut Oil and Milk

A coconut tree cannot produce both coconuts and coconut sugar. Coconut sugar, or the sap it is made from, is taken from the flower on the coconut palm tree, and the flower bud eventually forms a coconut. Many people are opposed to coconut sugar because of this. For this reason, I harbor a slight bias against it . . . but not enough to keep it out of my cocktails!

## 9. Coconut Xylose

As we saw in the previous item, there is some controversy surrounding the use of coconut sugar. Because of this, researchers are now making coconut xylose from coconut husks, which could be used as a sweetener. If this is successful, coconuts won't have to be sacrificed.

## 10. Which Side to Take?

Why do so many people believe that coconut sugar is more nutritious than other sugars? Because it is actually made from the sap that feeds the coconut flower, and this flower eventually grows to be a coconut bursting with so many health benefits.

# CHAPTER 9
# Ten Coconut Appetizers

*Thai Coconut Hummus*

### Ingredients

30-ounce can chickpeas, drained

3 garlic cloves

⅓ cup red curry paste

Zest of 2 limes

1 teaspoon salt

¾ cup unsweetened full-fat coconut milk, divided

Fresh Thai basil leaves as garnish

### Directions

Blend the chickpeas, garlic, red curry paste, and lime zest in a food processor. Season with the salt and add ½ cup of coconut milk.

Blend until the mixture is smooth. If it appears

that the hummus is too thick, mix in the remaining coconut milk.

Transfer the hummus to a serving bowl and garnish with Thai basil.

Serve with rice crackers or fresh vegetable sticks.

## *Coconut Bites*

### Ingredients
¼ cup coconut oil, solidified
½ cup coconut flour
2 tablespoons honey
Dash sea salt

### Directions
Preheat your oven to 350° F.

Combine the ingredients in a food processor. The mixture should be a bit sticky.

Use the mixture to form little balls.

Arrange the balls on an ungreased baking sheet and flatten the balls slightly.

Bake for about 10 minutes.

# Coconut Chips

## Ingredients
1 coconut
Coarse salt

## Directions
Preheat your oven to 350° F.

Pierce two eyes of the coconut, strain the water, and bake the coconut for half an hour. The shell may need more than 30 minutes to crack. Leave the coconut to cool until you can handle it.

To crack open the coconut, wrap it in a towel and hammer it several times. Split it into large pieces and separate the meat from the shell.

You can peel the dark outer skin or leave it if you wish. With a vegetable peeler or mandoline, make coconut strips, starting from the edges.

Scatter these strips on two baking sheets. Sprinkle the strips with salt and bake for about 10 minutes, until the coconut strips turn golden.

# Coconut Energy Bites

## Ingredients

¼ cup cashews

¾ cup almonds

1½ cups pitted medjool dates

Juice of 3 limes

Zest of 3 limes

Pinch of salt

⅓ cup unsweetened coconut flakes

## Directions

Pulse the cashews and almonds in a food processor until finely chopped. Blend in the dates, lime juice, and zest.

Make small balls from this mixture and roll them in the coconut flakes.

Store the balls in an airtight container and keep in the fridge.

## Stylish Shrimp Wontons

### Ingredients
Popcorn shrimp
Wonton wrappers
⅓ cup spicy chili dipping sauce
½ cup orange marmalade
⅓ cup sweetened coconut flakes
Coconut-oil spray

### Directions
Follow the package instructions to bake the popcorn shrimp.

In a bowl, whisk together the chili sauce and marmalade. Set aside.

Prepare your muffin pans by spraying them with coconut-oil spray. Use a wonton wrapper to line each muffin tin.

Add three pieces of baked shrimp to each muffin cup and top with a thin layer of marmalade and chili dip.

Sprinkle the wontons with coconut flakes, spray with coconut oil, and bake at 350° F for 5–7 minutes.

# Crunchy Coconut Apple Bites of Heaven

## Ingredients
1 apple, sliced into ¼-inch-thick slices
2 tablespoons coconut oil
2 tablespoons peanut butter
1 tablespoon dried cranberries
1 tablespoon chia seeds
1 teaspoon coconut flakes

## Directions
Assemble the apple bites on a plate and on each slice spread a layer of coconut oil and butter. Sprinkle the slices with cranberries, chia seeds, and coconut flakes.

# Nut Bites

## Ingredients
2 cups raw cashews
½ cup unsweetened peanut butter
2 cups medjool dates, pitted
2 tablespoons flax meal
¼ cup unsweetened coconut flakes

¼ teaspoon sea salt

3 tablespoons water

## Directions

Combine the cashews, peanut butter, and dates in a food processor.

Add the flax, coconut, and sea salt and process for a minute so that the mixture looks like crumbly dough. Finally, add the water to blend the ingredients.

Roll the mixture into small balls. Use a tablespoon as a measure.

Store the balls in the fridge.

## *Spirulina Coconutty Balls*

## Ingredients

1 cup chopped dates

1 cup raw pecan pieces

½ cup unsweetened raw coconut flakes

1 tablespoon spirulina

2 tablespoons coconut milk

2 tablespoons fresh lemon juice

2 tablespoons hemp seeds

### Directions

Chop the dates and pecans in a food processor. Add the remaining ingredients and blend until smooth.

Transfer the mixture to a bowl, cover it with plastic wrap, and put in the fridge.

After an hour or two, make small balls from this mixture. Use a teaspoon as a measure. Store the balls in an airtight container and keep them in the fridge.

## Coconut Peanut Dip

### Ingredients

1½ cups dry-roasted peanuts

4 tablespoons brown sugar

3 teaspoons red curry paste

1¼ cups coconut milk

3 tablespoons white wine vinegar

### Directions

In a small bowl, mix together the brown sugar and red curry. Set aside.

In a measuring cup, blend the vinegar and coconut milk. Set aside.

Blend the peanuts in a food processor until smooth. While processing the peanuts, add the curry and sugar mixture, and when it is incorporated, add the vinegar and coconut milk.

Process until the mixture is smooth.

Transfer to a serving bowl and serve with fresh vegetable sticks.

## Quick Deviled Eggs

**Ingredients**

1 dozen eggs, boiled and peeled

2 teaspoons rice vinegar

¼ cup peanut butter

1 tablespoon sugar

¾ teaspoon salt

½ teaspoon ginger powder

¼ teaspoon paprika

½ teaspoon cayenne pepper

½ teaspoon chili powder

3–4 tablespoons coconut milk

Coconut flakes to garnish

## Directions

Cut the boiled eggs in half. Scoop the yolks into a bowl and set the whites aside.

Blend the yolks with the vinegar, peanut butter, sugar, salt, and the spices until smooth.

Gradually pour in the coconut milk to get the texture of a mousse.

Fill the egg whites with this mixture. You can use a pastry bag for this.

Sprinkle the eggs with coconut flakes and serve at room temperature.

# CHAPTER 10

# Ten Coconut Entrees

*Slow-Cooker Coconut Quinoa Curry*

## Ingredients

1 large broccoli crown, cut into florets

½ white onion, diced

1 medium sweet potato, peeled and chopped

28 ounces canned coconut milk

28 ounces canned diced tomatoes

15 ounces canned organic chickpeas, drained and rinsed

2 garlic cloves, minced

¼ cup quinoa

1–1½ cups water

1 teaspoon chili flakes

1 teaspoon miso

2 teaspoons wheat-free tamari sauce

1 tablespoon freshly grated turmeric

1 tablespoon freshly grated ginger

### Directions

Combine the ingredients in your slow cooker.

    Set to high and cook for about 4 hours.

    Serve warm and enjoy!

## Chicken Gyro

### Ingredients

*For the tzatziki sauce*

1 can full-fat coconut milk

1 lemon, juiced

1 teaspoon grated garlic

4 tablespoons fresh dill, chopped

½ English cucumber, peeled and diced

Sea salt to taste

Ground black pepper to taste

NOTE: Refrigerate the coconut milk for at least 2 hours. The cream will separate from the liquid and float to the top.

*For the gyro wrap:*

4 tablespoons coconut flour

¾ cup tapioca starch

¼ teaspoon sea salt

1 cup full-fat organic coconut milk

2 eggs, whisked

2 tablespoons avocado oil or olive oil, divided

*For the chicken:*

1 tablespoon extra-virgin olive oil

2 cloves garlic, minced

2 lemons, 1 juiced and 1 sliced for garnish

½ teaspoon dried parsley

2 teaspoons dried oregano

½ teaspoon coriander

1 pound chicken breast

Sea salt to taste

Ground black pepper to taste

## Directions

*To prepare the tzatziki sauce:*

Combine the cream of the coconut milk with the other ingredients for the sauce.

Stir in the cucumber and place the sauce in the fridge until ready to serve.

*To prepare the gyro wrap:*

Mix together the coconut flour, tapioca flour, and salt.

In another bowl, whisk together the coconut milk, eggs, and a tablespoon of the oil.

Combine the wet and dry ingredients and mix well.

Heat the remaining oil in a skillet.

Divide the batter into 4 equal portions. Pour a portion into the skillet, flatten it, and fry until nicely browned on both sides.

Keep the wraps warm.

*To prepare the lemon chicken:*

Heat the oil in a skillet and sauté the minced garlic.

In a small bowl, combine all the remaining ingredients except the chicken.

Coat the chicken with this mixture and fry until cooked through.

To assemble the wrap, spread a layer of the tzatziki sauce over each gyro wrap, top with the chicken, and wrap them up.

# Lentil Coconut Curry

## Ingredients

1 cup crushed tomatoes

1 cup light coconut milk

1 tablespoon yellow curry paste

½ cup water

½ cup red lentils

¼ cup roasted, salted cashews

¼ cup packed fresh mint, roughly chopped

1 cup packed cilantro, roughly chopped

1 teaspoon jalapeño pepper, minced

½ teaspoon fresh ginger, minced

1 teaspoon fresh lime juice

2 tablespoons water

1 tablespoon coconut oil, melted

Salt and pepper, to taste

2 very large cucumbers, spiralized

## Directions

Combine the tomatoes, coconut milk, curry paste, and water. When it begins to boil, stir frequently, not allowing the mixture to form lumps.

Mix in the lentils and cook covered over low heat,

until the lentils absorb most of the liquid. This will take about 20 minutes.

In the meantime, blend the cashews in a food processor. Blend in the mint, cilantro, jalapeño pepper, ginger, and lime juice.

Gradually add the coconut oil and water while the processor is still running. The mixture should be creamy and smooth.

Use a paper towel to remove excess liquid from the spiralized cucumbers.

Transfer the cucumber "noodles" into a bowl and top them with the pesto. Toss to coat the noodles well.

Serve the noodles topped with the lentil curry.

## Chicken Curry

**Ingredients**
3 tablespoons virgin coconut oil
4 cloves garlic
¼ cup chopped onion
1 tablespoon curry powder
1 whole chicken, cut into 6–8 pieces

2 cups chicken stock

1 tablespoon chopped fresh ginger

½ teaspoon fine Himalayan salt

¼ teaspoon black pepper

2 tablespoons organic coconut flour

¼ cup water

## Directions

Heat the coconut oil and sauté the onion, garlic, and ginger.

Add the chicken and brown it on all sides.

Pour in the chicken stock and simmer for about 15 minutes.

Season with the black pepper, salt, and curry powder.

Cook covered for 5 more minutes.

In a small bowl, whisk the coconut flour and water and add it to the pan, stirring well.

Cook for 5 more minutes and serve warm over steamed rice.

## Salmon with Coconut Milk Sauce

### Ingredients

1 tablespoon fresh grated ginger

4 tablespoons coconut oil, divided

½ cup diced tomatoes

1 cup coconut milk

Salt and pepper, to taste

1 teaspoon coriander spice

4 salmon steaks

### Directions

Add the ginger and half of the coconut oil and heat for a minute. Add the tomatoes and cook for 3 to 5 minutes. Pour in the coconut milk and simmer covered over low heat for about 10 to 15 minutes.

Sprinkle the salmon steaks with salt, pepper, and coriander. Rub the mixture into the steaks.

Heat the remaining coconut oil in a grill pan.

Add the coconut sauce along with the salmon steaks. Cook the salmon for 5–7 minutes on each side, depending on how you want it done.

Serve the salmon with hot steaming rice and drizzled with the coconut sauce.

# Creamy Mushroom and Spinach Pasta

## Ingredients

1 package gluten-free spaghetti

2 cloves garlic, minced

1 can coconut milk

4 cups mushrooms, sliced

¼ teaspoon cayenne

Sea salt to taste

3 cups spinach

## Directions

Prepare the spaghetti following the package instructions. Set aside.

To prepare the sauce, combine the coconut milk with the mushrooms, garlic, cayenne, and sea salt.

Sauté over medium heat for 10–15 minutes.

Reduce heat to low and add the spaghetti and spinach. Stir well until the spinach has wilted.

Serve warm.

# Beef and Kale Stroganoff

## Ingredients
3 cups chopped kale, stems removed

10 ounces baby bella mushrooms, sliced

3 tablespoons butter, divided

1 teaspoon sea salt, divided

1½ pounds beef, cut into pieces

¾ cup beef stock

2 teaspoons yellow mustard

1 tablespoon tomato paste

½ teaspoon ground black pepper

½ cup full-fat coconut milk

1 tablespoon fresh chopped parsley

## Directions
Steam the kale until tender and set aside.

Melt a tablespoon of butter and sauté the mushrooms until brown. When done, season with salt, remove from the skillet, and set aside.

Add another tablespoon of butter, along with half the meat. Season with half the salt and leave the meat to brown nicely, and then stir it and cook for a minute or two. Remove from the pan and add to the mushrooms. Repeat with the remaining meat.

Add the stock to the hot pan and scrape the bits that are stuck to the bottom. Add the mustard, tomato paste, and black pepper.

Simmer for 5–10 minutes.

Stir in the coconut milk until incorporated. Add the mushrooms, kale, and meat and mix well.

Sprinkle with the parsley and serve hot.

## Coconut Chicken Fingers

**Ingredients**

3 chicken breasts, boneless and skinless, cut into long thin strips

1 teaspoon cayenne pepper

½ cup cornstarch

Salt and pepper to taste

3 eggs

2–3 cups sweetened coconut flakes

Oil for frying

**Directions**

Combine the cayenne pepper, cornstarch, pepper, and salt. Set aside.

In another bowl, beat the eggs and set aside.

Add the coconut flakes in another bowl.

Pour enough oil into a pot to fry the meat and heat it.

Coat the chicken in the cornstarch mixture, then drop the pieces in the bowl with the beaten eggs, and finally coat them with the shredded coconut.

When the oil is hot, fry the chicken pieces until cooked through and nicely golden. This will take about 3 minutes per side.

Place the fried chicken on a paper towel to get rid of any excess oil.

Serve with a spicy sauce of your choice.

## Kor-Lae Chicken

### Ingredients

16 dried chilies, soaked in warm water for 10 minutes

4 cups light coconut milk

3 pounds chicken thighs

6 ounces shallots

4 cups coconut cream

1 tablespoon coconut flour

2 tablespoons brown sugar

2 teaspoons salt

## Directions

Use the coconut milk to clean the chicken. Discard the milk and pat the chicken dry.

Using a blender, combine the shallots, coconut cream, and chilies. Transfer the mixture to a pan and heat over medium heat. Stir in the coconut milk and fry for about 2 minutes. Sprinkle with the brown sugar and salt.

Reserve a cup of this sauce and use the remaining sauce as a marinade for the chicken. Leave the chicken in this sauce overnight.

Preheat your oven to 350° F.

Heat the grill and sear the chicken for about 5 minutes per side, working in batches. When done, coat the chicken with the reserved sauce.

Finally, bake the chicken in the preheated oven for 10 minutes.

# Chickpea and Spinach Curry

## Ingredients

2 teaspoons olive oil

1 medium onion, finely chopped

1 teaspoon grated garlic

2 teaspoons minced ginger

¼ teaspoon cayenne pepper

½ teaspoon turmeric

2 cups chopped tomatoes

¾ teaspoon kosher salt

30 ounces canned low-sodium chickpeas, drained and
  rinsed

1 cup light coconut milk

2 teaspoons lemon juice

1 teaspoon garam masala

5 ounces baby spinach

Fresh cilantro for garnish

## Directions

Heat the oil in a pan, add the onion, and sauté for 5–7 minutes.

Stir in the garlic, ginger, cayenne, and turmeric, and cook for a minute until fragrant.

Stir in the tomatoes and season with salt.

Cook for 5–7 minutes, mashing the tomatoes into a puree using the back of a spoon. Pour in the coconut milk along with the chickpeas.

Leave the sauce to simmer until thickened.

Add the lemon juice and garam masala.

Add the spinach (do not stir it into the sauce) and cook for just a few minutes until the spinach has wilted.

Stir the spinach to coat it with the sauce. Garnish with the cilantro and serve hot with steamed rice or naan.

# Ten Coconut Desserts

## *Coconut Dark Chocolate Macaroons*

### Ingredients

¼ cup sugar

14½ ounces sweetened shredded coconut

½ teaspoon vanilla extract

½ cup sliced almonds

4 egg whites

½ teaspoon kosher salt

1⅔ cups raspberries

4 ounces dark chocolate

### Directions

Preheat your oven to 325° F. Line a baking sheet with parchment paper and set it aside.

In a food processor, blend the sugar, coconut, vanilla, almonds, egg whites, and salt. Mix in the raspberries.

Form balls from this mixture and arrange them on the prepared baking sheets.

Bake in the preheated oven for about half an hour. Leave the cookies to cool slightly.

Melt the chocolate, drizzle over the cookies, and leave to set before serving.

## Chocolate Coconut Candies

### Ingredients
1¾ cups flaked coconut
1¾ cups confectioners' sugar
½ cup sweetened condensed milk
1 cup chopped almonds
2 cups semisweet chocolate chips
2 tablespoons shortening

### Directions
Mix together the coconut, sugar, milk, and almonds. Use the mixture to form little balls.

Place the candies on a baking sheet and keep in the fridge for 20–30 minutes until hardened.

Melt the chocolate chips and shortening and dip the candies in the mixture to coat them.

Leave the candies on waxed paper until the chocolate has set.

## Piña Colada Cheesecake

**Ingredients**
1 cup flaked coconut, toasted
15 shortbread cookies, crushed
3 tablespoons butter, melted
*For the filling:*
¾ cup sugar
3 packages cream cheese
3 tablespoons 2% milk
¾ cup coconut cream
¾ teaspoon rum extract
3 eggs, lightly beaten
*For the topping:*
3 tablespoons apple jelly
½ fresh pineapple, peeled and cored

## Directions

Wrap a 9-inch springform pan with a double thickness of heavy-duty foil.

Mix together the coconut and cookie crumbs. Add the butter and blend well.

Transfer the mixture to the pan and press it into the bottom to form a crust.

Set this pan on a baking sheet and bake for 8–10 minutes at 325° F. Leave to cool.

Beat together the sugar and cream cheese. Mix in the milk, coconut, and rum extract. Beat in the eggs on low. Pour this cream over the cooled crust.

Place the pan in a larger pan that is filled with water to the depth of one inch.

Return to the oven and bake for one hour to one-and-a-half hours at 325° F.

Leave to cool. After about 10 minutes, run a knife around the edges of the cake. Leave to cool for one more hour and then keep in the fridge overnight.

Top the cheesecake with pineapple slices and brush them with warmed apple jelly.

# Golden Gem Cookies

## Ingredients

⅔ cup sugar

1 cup unsalted butter, room temperature

2 cups all-purpose flour

1 teaspoon salt

1 teaspoon vanilla extract

1½ cups sweetened shredded coconut flakes

1 egg beaten with 1 tablespoon water, for egg wash

1⅓ cups pineapple jam

## Directions

Use an electric mixer to combine the sugar and butter.

When the mixture gets fluffy, mix in the flour, salt, and vanilla. Wrap the bowl with plastic wrap and keep in the fridge for half an hour.

Preheat your oven to 350° F.

Use the dough to make little balls.

Roll the balls in the egg wash and then coat with coconut flakes. Make a small indentation in each cookie and fill it with the jam.

Bake for 20–25 minutes.

Leave to cool before serving.

# Coconut Triangles

## Ingredients

½ cup sweetened flaked coconut, toasted

6 tablespoons cornstarch

14 ounces coconut milk, divided

⅓ cup sugar

½ teaspoon vanilla

⅛ teaspoon salt

## Directions

Preheat your oven to 350° F.

Grease an 8-inch baking dish and set aside.

Combine ½ cup of coconut milk with the cornstarch. Set aside.

In a saucepan, mix together the remaining coconut milk and the sugar. Once the sugar has dissolved, add the cornstarch mixture and whisk along with the salt and vanilla.

Stir vigorously. Do not allow the mixture to boil. Cook for about 5 minutes, or until the mixture gets very thick.

Pour this cream into the baking dish and leave to cool.

Wrap it with plastic wrap and keep in the fridge for an hour.

Cut into triangles or squares and sprinkle with toasted coconut.

## *Strawberry and Coconut Bars*

**Ingredients**

½ cup butter, melted

1⅔ cups graham cracker crumbs

2⅔ cups flaked coconut

1 cup strawberry preserves

14 ounces sweetened condensed milk

⅓ cup chopped walnuts, toasted

¼ cup white baking chips

½ cup semisweet chocolate chips

**Directions**

Mix the butter and cracker crumbs. Add this mixture to a greased baking dish. Press the mixture into the bottom to make a crust.

Bake for about 20 minutes at 350° F. Leave to cool.

Top the crust with the strawberry preserves and walnuts.

Melt the chocolate chips and coat the walnuts.

Melt the white chips as well, and drizzle over the cake.

Leave to harden. Cut into bars and place in the fridge for half an hour.

## *Toasted Coconut Ice Cream*

**Ingredients**

2 cups sweetened coconut, toasted

2 cups cream

1 cup whole milk

6 egg yolks

¾ cup sugar

2 teaspoons grated lime zest

½ teaspoon kosher salt

**Directions**

In a saucepan, combine the toasted coconut with milk and cream. When it begins to boil, stir well, cover, and set aside for an hour.

In another saucepan, combine the sugar and egg yolks and cook until the mixture has thickened slightly.

Strain the coconut mixture and add it slowly to the egg mixture. Whisk continuously until well combined. Cook over medium heat until it turns into custard. Make sure to stir frequently.

Strain the custard and pour into an airtight container. Mix in the salt and lime zest.

Chill overnight, and then follow the manufacturer's instructions for your ice cream maker to make the ice cream.

Keep the ice cream in an airtight container and freeze for 4 hours before serving.

## Coconut Angel Pie

**Ingredients**
1 pastry shell, baked
¼ cup cornstarch
½ cup sugar
2 cups whole milk
¼ teaspoon salt

3 egg yolks, lightly beaten

1 tablespoon butter

½ cup flaked coconut

1½ teaspoons vanilla extract

*For the meringue:*

¼ teaspoon cream of tartar

3 egg whites

¼ teaspoon vanilla extract

6 tablespoons sugar

¼ cup flaked coconut

## Directions

In a saucepan, combine the cornstarch, sugar, and salt, and place over medium heat. Stir in the milk and cook until the mixture has thickened. Reduce the heat and cook for 2 more minutes, stirring continuously.

Remove the saucepan from the heat. Take a small amount of the mixture and add it to the egg yolks.

Pour this into the saucepan and return to the stove.

When it begins to boil, cook for 2 more minutes, stirring continuously.

Remove from the stove once again and add the butter, coconut, and vanilla. Mix well.

Transfer the mixture to the prepared shell.

Use an electric mixer to beat the cream of tartar, egg whites, and vanilla. Gradually add in sugar and then spread the mixture over the hot cream.

Sprinkle with the coconut and bake for about 20 minutes at 350° F.

Leave to cool for about an hour and then place in the fridge for 3–4 hours before serving.

## Coconut Hot Chocolate

### Ingredients
28 ounces sweetened condensed milk

4 13-ounce cans full-fat coconut milk

8 ounces high-quality dark chocolate, chopped

¼ teaspoon salt

¼ cup Dutch process cocoa powder

2 teaspoons coconut extract

2 teaspoons vanilla extract

½ cup unsweetened flaked coconut

Marshmallows for topping

Whipped cream for topping

## Directions

In a crockpot, combine the condensed milk, coconut milk, and extracts.

Add the cocoa powder, salt, and chocolate, and mix well.

Cover, set on low, and cook for 2 hours.

Make sure to stir the mixture every 15 minutes.

When serving, rim the mug edges with glazing and then dip them into toasted coconut flakes. Fill the mugs with chocolate and top with marshmallows and whipped cream.

## *Coconut and Banana Ice Cream*

### Ingredients

1 tablespoon lemon juice

6 very ripe medium bananas, peeled

¾ cup light corn syrup

1 cup coconut milk

1 tablespoon dark rum

¼ cup virgin coconut oil

¼ teaspoon kosher salt

## Directions

Combine the lemon juice and bananas in a food processor. While the processor is still running, gradually add the corn syrup, coconut, rum, coconut oil, and salt.

Strain this mixture and press plastic wrap across its surface.

Keep in the fridge for about 4 hours.

Use this mixture to make ice cream following the manufacturer's instructions for your ice cream maker.

Store in an airtight container and keep in the freezer for at least 3 hours before serving.

# CHAPTER 12

# Ten Coconut Drinks

## *Coconut Beach*

### Ingredients

1 cup ice

½ ounce Frangelico

1 ounce coconut rum

1 ounce white rum

3 tablespoons dairy-free coconut ice cream

Toasted coconut flakes

### Directions

Blend the ingredients in your blender until smooth.

Fill your serving glasses, sprinkle with the toasted coconut, and serve.

## Cocoa Bliss Smoothie

### Ingredients
½ cup full-fat coconut milk

1 cup almond milk

1 teaspoon no-alcohol pure vanilla

1 tablespoon coconut butter

1 tablespoon cocoa powder

### Directions
Combine the ingredients in a blender until smooth. Serve and enjoy.

## Piña Coladas

### Ingredients
2 ounces coconut milk

6–8 ounces rum (optional)

1 large mango

5 cups diced pineapple

2 cups ice

## Directions

To prepare the mango, peel it and remove the seed.

Dice the mango and set aside a few pieces for garnish. Puree the remaining diced mango until smooth and set aside.

To prepare the piña colada, combine the coconut milk, pineapple, and ice. Once the mixture is smooth, add the rum. Mix in a spoonful of the mango puree.

Fill one-third of each serving glass with this mixture. Add a spoonful of the mango puree and swirl again.

Fill the glasses two-thirds full with piña colada and swirl in a spoonful of the mango puree.

Top each glass with the remaining piña colada and the reserved diced mango.

## *Coconut Margarita*

### Ingredients

8 ounces coconut water

3 ounces tequila blanco

3 ounces light coconut milk

1½ ounces triple sec

Lime wedges, for serving

Ice, for serving

### Directions

Shake together the tequila blanco, coconut milk, coconut water, and triple sec.

Place a few ice cubes in each serving glass. Fill the glasses with the cocktail. Garnish with lime wedges and serve.

## Banana Piña Colada

### Ingredients

1 banana, peeled, frozen, and sliced

1 cup vanilla soy milk

3 ounces coconut rum

½ cup crushed pineapple

### Directions

Add the ingredients in a blender and combine until smooth.

Pour into a glass and enjoy!

# Coconut Rum Slushie

## Ingredients

1½ cups crushed ice

3 tablespoons coconut rum

3 tablespoons frozen limeade concentrate

Lime wedge, for garnish

## Directions

Combine the ingredients (except for the lime wedges) in a blender until the mixture gets slushy.

Serve in a glass garnished with a lime wedge.

# Coconut Banana Shake

## Ingredients

⅔ cup canned unsweetened coconut milk

1 container vanilla coconut milk yogurt

¼ cup Nutella

2 frozen bananas, peeled and sliced

¼ teaspoon ground clove

¼ teaspoon ground ginger

¼ teaspoon ground cardamom

¼ teaspoon ground cinnamon

Coconut flakes for garnish

### Directions

Add the ingredients in a blender and combine until smooth.

Pour in glasses, sprinkle with coconut flakes, and serve.

## Spicy Coconut Agua Fresca

### Ingredients

*For the Chile de Arbol Syrup:*

1 cup sugar

1 cup water

5 dried chiles de arbol, torn

*For the Agua Fresca:*

1 cup coconut water

2 pounds whole honeydew melon

1 tablespoon fresh lime juice

1 tablespoon chile de arbol simple syrup

Fresh melon for garnish (optional)

## Directions

*To prepare the Chile de Arbol Syrup:*

Combine the sugar and water in a saucepan. Add the torn chilies and bring to a boil. Stir the mixture and reduce heat to simmer.

Cook for about 10 minutes and then remove from the heat and leave to cool.

Strain the liquid and keep it in the fridge.

*To prepare the Agua Fresca:*

Puree the honeydew in a blender. Strain the puree by pouring it into a colander lined with cheesecloth.

Leave to strain for about 10 minutes. Squeeze to extract any remaining juice.

Combine 1½ cups of this juice with the chile de arbol syrup, coconut water, and lime juice.

Keep in the fridge before serving. Serve chilled and garnished with cubes of fresh honeydew melon.

## *Tropical Water*

### Ingredients

½ cup pure coconut water

¾ cup fresh pineapple juice

1 teaspoon honey

½ teaspoon pure ginger juice

1 lime

### Directions

If you don't have a shaker, use a mason jar to combine the coconut water, pineapple juice, and ginger juice.

Add some ice.

Shake and taste. If you want it a bit sweeter, add some honey.

Fill the glasses with ice cubes and lime slices. Pour in the coconut and pineapple concoction and serve.

## Wild Smoothie

### Ingredients

6 fluid ounces coconut milk

1 cup fresh pineapple

1¼ cup frozen wild blueberries

1 teaspoon chia seeds

1 tablespoon fresh mint leaves, torn

## Directions

Place the ingredients in a blender and combine until smooth. Serve and enjoy!

# Conclusion

And so you have come to the end of this coconut journey. It's been an amazing adventure, starting from the very first coconuts, followed by their colonization of the world. Due to their numerous health benefits and uses, coconuts can be found in various forms. And in case you got curious about what coconuts have to offer, you can enjoy the coconut recipes from this book and surprise your taste buds with tropical coconut flavors that are bursting with health!

# Bibliography

"A Brief Look at the History of Coconuts," accessed February 2016, http://www.be-healthy-with-coconuts.com/history-of-coconuts.html.

Asaff, B. "Is a Coconut a Nut or a Fruit?" http://vegetarian.lovetoknow.com/Is_a_Coconut_a_Nut.

Asprey, D. "5 Not-So-Sweet Facts about Coconut Sugar," accessed February 28, 2016, https://www.bulletproofexec.com/5-not-so-sweet-facts-about-coconut-sugar/.

Assunção, M. L. et al. "Effects of Dietary Coconut Oil on the Biochemical and Anthropometric Profiles of Women Presenting Abdominal Obesity," *Lipids* 44 no. 7 (2009): 593–601.

Bernard, J. "Nutrition in Coconut Sugar," last modified May 23, 2015, accessed February 19, 2016, http://www.livestrong.com/article/540370-nutrition-in-coconut-sugar/.

"Biofuel," accessed February 20, 2016, http://www.kokonutpacific.com.au/Coconut-BiofuelKP.php#continued.

Bonneau, X. et al. "Coconut Husk Ash as a Fertilizer for Coconut Palms on Peat," *Experimental Agriculture* 46 no. 3 (2010): 401–414.

Brown, D. "7 More Reasons to Drink Coconut Water," last modified April 4, 2015, accessed February 18, 2016, http://www.mindbodygreen.com/0-18146/7-more-reasons-to-drink-coconut-water.html.

Campbell-Falck, D. et al. "The Intravenous Use of Coconut Water," *American Journal of Emergency Medicine* 18 no. 1 (2000): 108–11.

Cimons, M. "Company Converts Coconut Husk Fibers into Materials for Cars and Homes," last modified July 23, 2014, accessed February 21, 2016, http://phys.org/news/2014-07-company-coconut-husk-fibers-materials.html.

"Coconets," last modified April 27, 2012, accessed February 20, 2016, http://www.aljazeera.com/programmes/ earthrise/ 2012/04/ 201242715330787850.html

"Coconut Info: History, Origin and Properties," accessed February 27, 2016, http://www.coconut-info.net/.

"Coconut Oil Could Combat Tooth Decay," last modified September 3, 2012, accessed February 21, 2016, BBC, http://www.bbc.com/news/health-19435442.

"Coconut Palm Sugar. The Truth about Coconut Palm Sugar: The Other Side of the Story!" accessed February 28, 2016, https://www.tropicaltraditions.com/coconut_palm_sugar.htm.

"Coconut Palm Trees—Interesting Facts about Them," accessed February 15, 2016, http://www.coconut-info.net/general/coconut_trees.php.

"Coconut Palm," accessed February 28, 2016, Encyclopædia Britannica Online, http://www.britannica.com/plant/coconut-palm.

"Coconut Secrets for Optimal Health," accessed February 28, 2016, https://www.coconutsecret.com/coconuthealthsecrets2.html.

"Coconut Water Nutrition Facts," accessed February 28,

2016, http://www.nutrition-and-you.com/coconut-water.html.

"Coconuts and Its Secrets—Part I," accessed February 18, 2016, http://www.ecellulitis.com/skin-health/coconuts-and-its-secrets-part-i/.

Costantini, L. et al. "Hypometabolism as a Therapeutic Target in Alzheimer's Disease," *BMC Neuroscience* 9 no. 2 (2008): S16.

Dansereau, A. "The Numerous Health Benefits of Coconuts," last modified August 22, 2012, accessed February 15, 2016, http://www.care2.com/greenliving/the-numerous-health-benefits-of-coconuts-2.html.

Dreon, D. M. et al. "Change in Dietary Saturated Fat Intake Is Correlated with Change in Mass of Large Low-Density-Lipoprotein Particles in Men," *American Journal of Clinical Nutrition* 67 no. 5 (1998): 828–836.

Elsass, P. "What Are the Benefits of Coconut Vinegar?" last modified April 23, 2015, accessed February 27, 2016, http://www.livestrong.com/article/262961-what-are-the-benefits-of-coconut-vinegar/

Gunn, B. F. et al. "Independent Origins of Cultivated Coconut (Cocos nucifera L.) in the Old World Tropics," *PLoS ONE* 6 no. 6 (2011): e21143 DOI:10.1371/journal.pone.0021143.

Gunnars, K. "10 Proven Health Benefits of Coconut Oil (No. 3 Is Best)," last modified February, 2016, accessed February 21, 2016, http://authoritynutrition.com/top-10-evidence-based-health-benefits-of-coconut-oil/.

Gunnars, K. "Coconut Sugar—Healthy Sugar Alternative

or a Big, Fat Lie?" last modified November, 2015, accessed February 20, 2016, http://authoritynutrition.com/coconut-sugar/.

"Health Benefits of Coconut Oil," accessed February 27, 2016, https://www.organicfacts.net/health-benefits/oils/health-benefits-of-coconut-oil.html.

Icasas, P. "10 Awesome Facts about Coconuts," last modified August 28, 2013, accessed February 18, 2016, http://listverse.com/2013/08/28/10-awesome-facts-about-coconuts/.

"Is a Coconut a Fruit, Nut or Seed?" accessed February 19, 2016, The Library of Congress, http://www.loc.gov/rr/scitech/mysteries/coconut.html.

"Is Coconut a Fruit or a Nut?" accessed February 17, 2016, http://www.thebestofrawfood.com/is-coconut-a-fruit.html.

Lee, C. "Can Coconuts Help You Lose Weight?" last modified August 26, 2014, accessed February 19, 2016, http://www.bewellfx.com/be-nourished/2014/8/21/are-coconuts-just-a-product-of-a-food-trend.

Lewin, J. "The Health Benefits of . . . Coconut Milk," BBC Good Food, accessed February 28, 2016, http://www.bbcgoodfood.com/howto/guide/ingredient-focus-coconut-milk.

Lutz, D. "Deep History of Coconuts Decoded," Washington University in Saint Louis, last modified June 24, 2011, accessed February 20, 2016, https://source.wustl.edu/2011/06/deep-history-of-coconuts-decoded/.

Maravilla, J. N. and Magat, S. S. "Sequential Coconut

Toddy (Sap) and Nut Production (SCTNP) in Laguna Tall Variety and Hybrid Coconuts," *Philipp. J. Crop Science* 18 no. 3 (1993): 143–152.

Martin A. "8 Benefits of Coconut Water You Didn't Know About," accessed February 28, 2016, http://www.lifehack.org/articles/lifestyle/8-benefits-coconut-water-you-didnt-know-about.html.

McClernon, F. J. et al. "The Effects of a Low-Carbohydrate Ketogenic Diet and a Low-Fat Diet on Mood, Hunger, and Other Self-Reported Symptoms," *Obesity (Silver Spring)* 15 no. 1 (2007): 182–187.

Nevin, K. G. and Rajamohan, T. "Influence of Virgin Coconut Oil on Blood Coagulation Factors, Lipid Levels and LDL Oxidation in Cholesterol Fed Sprague–Dawley Rats," *European e-Journal of Clinical Nutrition and Metabolism* 3 no. 1 (2008): e1–e8.

Noor, S. F. "Unique Uses of Coconut," last modified July 8, 2015, accessed February 17, 2016, http://www.boldsky.com/home-n-garden/decor/2015/unique-uses-of-coconut-075786.html.

Phan, N. "Ketogenic Diet as a Treatment for Refractory Epilepsy," *Journal on Developmental Disabilities* 13 no. 3 (2007): 189–204.

"Raw, Virgin, Unrefined, Organic, Expeller-Pressed Coconut Oil—Which Is Best?" last modified February 25, 2009, http://kellythekitchenkop.com/raw-virgin-unrefined-organic-expeller-pressed-coconut-oil-which-is-best/.

Saxelby, C. "Coconut Sugar," last modified December 10, 2014, accessed February 21, 2016, http://foodwatch.com.au/blog/carbs-sugars-and-fibres/

item/coconut-sugar.html.

Shilhavy, B. and Shilhavy, M. "Coconut Oil Benefits for Digestive Health," accessed February 29, 2016, http://healthimpactnews.com/2012/coconut-oil-benefits-for-digestive-health/.

"The Coconut Husk Is a Cutting Edge Technology," accessed February 27, 2016, http://www.be-healthy-with-coconuts.com/coconut-husk.html.

"The Kitavan Diet: Tubers, Fresh Fruit, Coconut and Fish," accessed February 19, 2016, http://www.healwithfood.org/diet/kitavan-diet-foods.php#ixzz41TyA18hu.

"Treating Eczema and Psoriasis with Coconut and Other Natural Oils," last modified October 3, 2015, accessed February 22, 2016, http://homeremediesforlife.com/coconut-oil-for-eczema/.

Ward, D. and English, J. "Beneficial Effects on Energy, Atherosclerosis and Aging," Nutritionre, last modified April 22, 2013, accessed February 23, 2016, http://nutritionreview.org/2013/04/medium-chain-triglycerides-mcts/.

Zelman, K. M. "The Truth about Coconut Water," accessed February 28, 2016, http://www.webmd.com/food-recipes/truth-about-coconut-water.

# About the Author

Some people say that Morgan H. Bishop was born beneath a palm tree and weaned on coconut milk. However, the truth is more likely that he was conceived after copious consumption of piña coladas. This legendary writer has had a lifelong obsession with the regal coconut, which has driven him to serious scientific inquiry and countless hours of contemplation and experimentation with all facets of the fruit, starting with the palm tree. This book marks his first attempt to share his findings with the world.

Morgan H. Bishop has multiple manuscripts in the works and spends the majority of his time freelancing, often as a ghostwriter. You will soon find more of his work floating around in cyberspace.

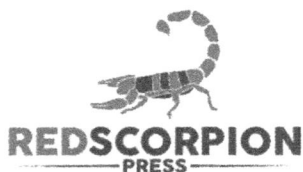

**REDSCORPION**
— PRESS —

Red Scorpion Press was formed in January 2016 with the hope of bettering the world in a small way through publishing. Our aim is to push boundaries and be an outlet for fresh voices and unique perspectives that entertain and inform.

Please visit us at www.redscorpionpress.com for our latest selection of books.